VEGAN BOOK

Why Becoming Vegan Can Be Dangerous to Your Health and How to Do It Right

Introduction

In the early 1860s, the very first form of diet was introduced to the public. It was conceived by an English coffin-maker, William Banting, from whom the name of the diet was taken. *Banting* required cutting the intake of starch and sugary carbs in the food we eat every day. This includes cutting six ounce of meat, as well, and washing everything down with a good glass of claret.

It might sound cliché, but we are *exactly* what we eat, and it will show in many ways; from the way our hair shines, the way our eyes glisten, the redness of our lips, and even the radiance of our skin. Still, a lot of us do not pay attention to what we eat and how beneficial proper diet is.

According to a recent health report released by *The Organisation for Economic Co-operation and Development (OECD)*, "more than one in two adults and nearly one in six children are overweight or obese." Moreover, United States still ranked first in the countries with highest obesity rate in the world, followed by Mexico, New Zealand, and Hungary. The lowest being Japan and Korea.

However, since the conception of the Banting diet, many other diet practices came about in books and leaflets, and the list just skyrocketed since then. Each diet proposes a certain amount of food to take, dietary benefits, and a specific exercise that comes with it. Each diet, whilst promising, are geared up towards one goal: to have a healthy lifestyle that can get you pass the 80-year-old life expectancy mark.

This book will discuss one specific diet, which has been in practice long before Banting was even introduced. This diet goes back to when the earliest form of men still roam the face of the earth. This book will also help you prepare for this type of diet and lifestyle by giving you guides on how to make the transition from your current lifestyle and making sumptuous meals vegan style.

Chapter One: The Concept of Veganism

1.a Vegetarianism vs. Veganism

Vegetarianism is the practice of cutting meat consumption by a large percentage in every meal we take. Exceptions are made here and there, as some would still eat dairy and egg products.

Veganism is a philosophical concept of abstaining or removing anything that involves the exploitation of animals from the human practice and system; from the food we eat, the products we use, and the clothes we wear, and by extension, promulgates the conservation of animal welfare and promotes animal-free alternatives for both human beings and environment.

Introduced in 1944 by Donald Watson when he co-founded the Vegan Society in England, the term *vegan* became widely accepted by those who follow the philosophy or the practice of it, or both as he believed that vegetarianism is often confused with veganism. The society filtered the early definition of veganism to "the doctrine that man should live without exploiting animals."

There are several types of vegans. This is because vegans have different patterns that they follow which can be categorized according to the following:

Vegans (total vegetarians): People who do not eat anything that has meat from any animals.

Lacto-ovo vegetarians: People who do not eat meat, with the exception of eggs and diary products.

Lacto vegetarians: People who do not eat any meat at all, saved from dairy products.

Ovo vegetarians: People who do not eat meat, but eat eggs.

Partial vegetarians: Avoid meat but may eat fish (pesco-vegetarian, pescatarian) or poultry (pollo-vegetarian).

There are a lot of reasons why a person chooses a vegan lifestyle. One reason is, according to an article released by Harvard Health Publication, a large number of the population chooses vegan diet because they can't afford meat. A normal grocery bag of an average American would normally include broccoli, potatoes, carrots, apples, banana, and can tomatoes. Other obvious reasons include health, religious convictions, and concern about animal welfare, However, the year-round availability of fresh produce, green leafy vegetarian dining alternatives and the growing fascination towards Asian cuisines can be some of the main reasons why people choose vegan diet.

As mentioned previously, Japan and Korea ranked the least with obese people in their countries. Asian countries are known for their low-fat healthy eating lifestyle which gives emphasis to green leafy vegetables, fresh fruits and very little to none meat. With 3:1 vegetable meat ratio, dietitians and researchers believe that this specific lifestyle contributes to the Asian community's longevity in life expectancy.

1.b The Asian Way of Vegan

It's true that we are what we eat. It's not just a saying that makes us rethink that way we see food and its benefits, but it's also a philosophy. And there is no better way of explaining this thru examples than by looking into a largely practiced diet in Asia.

Asians have a long-standing customs, which is often closely tied with traditions and religious practices. These customs are also the main inspiration and practical source for culinary alternatives.

The Asian Diet Pyramid is an infographic that illustrates Asian Diet. The pyramid was developed to illustrate a careful discipline for healthy living. This, as a result, gives us an insight towards historical low records of chronic diseases and other health-related issues on a specific region/country. The Asian Diet's geographical base is very broad. It includes (but is not limited to) Bangladesh, Cambodia, China, India, Indonesian, Japan, Laos, Malaysia, Mongolia, Myanmar, Nepal, North Korea, South Korea, Philippines, Singapore, Taiwan, Thailand, and Vietnam.

The constant members of the Asian diet pyramid are vegetable and tubers, fruits, grains, nuts, seeds, legumes, herbs and spices. Now, this does not mean Asians are so tied with these fresh produce because they can't afford meat as what was written in the Harvard Health Publication. Asians can afford meat, even the average Asian family can afford salmon, and tuna, which are sold at a high price in the U.S. Conclusively, Asians have deep-seated practice of being practical in almost all aspects of their lives. But they've also mastered the art of getting much from spending so little, and this practice is very evident in the way they prepare their meals.

It is also imperative to remember that Asians do not just rely on eating low fat and fresh produce meals. They couple it with proper exercises such as yoga, jogging and even the simplest exercise available: walking.

1.c The American Adaptation of Vegan Diet

To start with, the West did no catch on in the rise of vegan as much as Europe did. It was not until the early 1900s when Americans realized the growing number of chronic heart diseases, diabetes, cancer, and obesity, which are all linked to one thing: poor diet.

According to an article published thru Huffington Post, today, more Americans are aware of the vegetarian-based diet. In 2012, meat consumption was cut down by 12.2 percent, and it is estimated that half of the American population is now aware of the 'Meatless Monday' practice; more are observing eating at least one vegetarian meal in a week.

Startling to believe but more and more Americans are now eating meals that has little to none fish, meat, or poultry in it; several millions have completely eradicated red meat from their grocery bags. Quoting again from the report released by

Harvard Health Publications, "about two million have become vegans, forgoing not only animal flesh but also animal-based products such as milk, cheese, eggs, and gelatin."

However, what does this tell us? It can be inferred that Americans are now starting to see the benefits of a vegetarian-based diet, more or less, the same way their Asian neighbors does. This resulted to a rise of vegan alternatives on the market, in fact in 2013, American supermarket saw a paradigm shift in terms of the top food trends. New vegetarian and vegetarian proteins replaced common meat commodities and over 100 meat substitutes were introduced.

Restaurants are the major players in this shift in the demand from meat to no-meat meals. The food industry in the United States also saw a shift in the way meals are prepared. The successful penetration of the vegan items in the traditional menus and recipes suggest not only the change in our attitude towards the food we eat but also on the type of diet we have, which is essential for health care providers and pharmaceutical companies on the long run.

Chapter Two: Things You Need To Know

2a. 16 Tips To Consider Before Going Vegan

Now that you know what Vegan is and why is there such a craze about it, to the extent that it increased demands for vegan alternatives and caused paradigm shifts in both producer-consumer relationships, it's time to know how to make the transition.

There are a few things that a vegan-want-to-be needs to know. It is imperative that one needs to know how to properly transition from his or her current lifestyle to a vegan lifestyle. There are people who do the transition overnight and often this leads to health problems.

Like any other transitions in life, making the vegan transition requires time, dedication, and total commitment. It's definitely something that can't be achieved overnight. Below are collated information from experts about this field. These are things that you need to know before making this lifestyle change.

1. **Plan a Gradual Transition**

    Studies show that gradual transitions result to people sticking to it rather than doing it haphazardly or overnight.

You can start cutting animal-based meal slowly, especially if you a diet fairly heavy in meat. It would also be advisable to seek professional advice from doctors or dietitian to assist you with a diet calendar and menus.

2. **One Step at a Time**

   Hype of something drives us to want to make things happen with a snap. But if this concerns your health, doctors would say no to magic. Just like doing exercises at the gym for a specific goal, it is highly advisable to make a transition from meat-full diet to vegan one-step at a time. Again, small changes per day will result to a long-term dedication and better result. It really doesn't matter when you're going to feel fully adjusted to the new diet since there's no timeline. You can totally take your time for as long as the end goal will be you adapting the vegan diet.

3. **Balance Small Changes with Big Changes**

   So you've finally managed to eradicate meat from your meals, and that's a good thing. The adjustment period is pass your way and it was a lot of effort to put in to. Then a friend invited you for a barbeque one Sunday. The dilemma is something you didn't hope for. In actuality, there's nothing to worry about; instead of mulling over cancelling, you can consider a lot of alternatives like asking for a vegan option, which they'll surely have. There's no need to make a sweeping change when you can make small tweaks along the way.

4. **Follow What's Best For You**

   There's a lot of perpetual listicles on the internet about how to transition from fairly heavy meat diet to vegan diet and it can be very overwhelming. And since it's proven to be overwhelming, you just choose one source and try to follow it religiously, including those items in the list that are proving to be difficult. Experts suggest that you should follow what you can only follow and do not push yourself to much. (*Refer to item 2: One Step at a Time*). Again, the important thing in making the transition is it works to your advantage and not the other way around.

5. **Going Vegan is Not Equivocal to Going to the Gym**

   This is a common misconception that *everyone* needs to be mindful of. Again, there is a plethora of reasons why a person goes vegan, one of which being for health reasons. Many people as well think that if they go vegan, they will magically lose weight. Let it be clear that going vegan *can contribute* to weight loss. Daily and proper exercises are still top options to lose weight, proper diet comes next.

6. **Expect for Cheat Days Along The Way**

   Routines are very demanding, we all get that. We put in so much effort into something at times that we also get tired of doing it. That is the reason why cheat days are also expected every now and then. But this is okay, for as long as you have to come back on track and never stop.

7. **Eat More Beans**

   Beans are great source of protein and fiber and is perfect as dietary staple for those making the transition to vegan diet. One can never go wrong with this humble crop.

   Protein is one of the most important minerals that our body needs. According to WedMD, protein is responsible for our body's production of enzymes, hormones, and other body chemicals. Protein is also beneficial in maintaining body tissues, building our bones, muscles, cartilages, skin and blood.

8. **Take it Easy on Dietary Restrictions**

   Unless you've been told to do so by a doctor or dietitian, there's no need to further cut down something from your diet as you make the transition to vegan-based diet. Doing so will only make the transition restrictive and hard to follow.

9. **Build Your Vegan Circle**

Sharing can be a source of mutual support and it has proven to be effective in maintaining a practice or a new routine. To make the transition a lot easier and fun, experts advise to surround yourself with fellow vegan friends, or find one online. Not only you can share this close familiarity, you can also share and exchange your diet palates and menus.

10. **Locate Restaurants and Cafes That Offer Vegan Alternatives**

A lot of us live in a fast-phase working environment and in between making that report for a scheduled meeting, meeting a client, and finishing other industry-related work, finding a place where vegan-based diet is being offered can be challenging at times. Advise: locate ahead of time near-by restaurants and cafes that offer vegan alternatives and you will be good.

11. Vegan Desert Check

In the event that you find yourself in a vegan restaurant, Chinese, Thai, Ethiopian and Indian vegan diet are great options. In terms of desert, it will never hurt to ask for tofu.

12. Learn The Art of Cooking

There is no easy way to be vegan, that's for sure. Therefore, you have to master a few arts that comes with it, to include cooking. You have to learn how to cook for yourself and cook vegan-based diet. This is proven effective, cost-efficient, and handy especially if you are invited for dinner parties.

13. Ask The Chef

Just in case you find yourself in an awkward situation where there is no vegan alternative on the menu, feel free to ask if the chef can whip you up a salad with beans and grilled vegetables. Fries can also be a good alternative.

14. Take Vitamin B12

The natural source for vitamin B12 is, unfortunately, in animal-based food. Experts are strict enough on this that vegans should take vitamin B12 supplements to augment the need. According to experts — Ginny Messina, registered dietician, and Ryan Andrews, registered dietician — though you can get some B12 in fortified foods like plant milks and veggie meats, to get as much as you need, a supplement is essential.

15. Be Mindful of Weird Changes

According to the article published thru BuzzFeed, Both Messina and Andrews say that eating well, being healthy, and feeling great are possible for almost anyone eating a healthy, varied, whole foods-based vegan diet. Nevertheless, if you notice some weird changes like fatigue, lack of sleep, or you just feel off at times while working out, you need to tweak some of your diet routines and seek for experts' advice. Remember, what might work for others may not work for you.

16. Know What The Experts Say

It is imperative to know what the experts have to say in making this transition. The internet can be a great source of materials in matters like this but the internet is not a medical expert. It wouldn't hurt you to ask the right source, would it?

2b. Why Becoming Vegan Can Be Dangerous to Your Health?

Registered nutritionists suggest that as we try to make drastic lifestyle changes, there are negative sides that come along with it. Deciding to follow an all-plant based diet could help lose those fats quickly; some medical experts say that this could also post health-related risks.

Lily Soutter is a registered nutritional therapist at the Institute of Optimum Nutrition, and regularly write articles for The Times, The Telegraph, The Independent, The Daily Mail, Cosmopolitan and Women's Health. She revealed stunning pitfalls of following a vegan-based diet.

"It is possible to eliminate animal products and still have a nutritionally adequate diet," Lily said in one article published by The Daily Mail.

She mentioned that transitioning from a meat-full diet to a plant-based diet should be planned carefully as there are factors that need to be considered so as not to "succumb to the nutritional deficiencies that can often come alongside a vegan diet."

She highlighted that cutting meat intake from your palate means cutting down essential vitamins that can naturally be acquired from animal-based products, and this can result to deficiencies. Moreover, Lily explained that deficiencies could result to fatigue, megaloblastic anaemia, early dementia, increased risk of heart disease, nerve dysfunction, forgetfulness, lack of coordination and psychiatric disorder.

In stark comparison, plant-based diet has small content of omega 3 oils. This means you your source of vegan alternative should have enough oil to augment the lack of omega 3, which is naturally present in oily fish.

Much of the health-related concerns that make vegan diet alarming for some is the apparent lack of minerals that the body needs. But experts says that for as long as one can augment these deficiencies and be able to look for a vegan-diet that works best for them, everything should be fine. Chapter 3 will cover preparations for going vegan and recipes that can be prepared to jump-start your vegan lifestyle the safe way.

2c. Simple Tips to Get You Started the Right Way

Previous chapters talk about what veganism is and what you need to know. One recurring theme, however, which is very important, is getting it planned the right way This section will give you some talking points and questions to answer to jump start your "planning" in becoming a vegan.

1. **Proper mindset**

   Mindset is important in anything because it psyches you to engage into something. Having proper mindset about this transition is very important now that you know the do's and don'ts of becoming a vegan. This will enable your mind to engage your senses in making this transition. An important reminder is to never rush and pressure yourself in doing this. Also, just because you are doing vegan it automatically means you're 100 percent healthy. Still, you have to do exercises.

2. **Engage Your Family and Friends**

   Announce your plan to the world not because you want to show off but you need support in doing so. Your family and friends will play a vital role in this transition. This way, they will be given heads up and will be able to help you along the way by means of meals to offer and prepare in certain occasions.

3. **Carefully Plan Your Menu**

You need to make researches on vegan meals that are applicable for breakfast, lunch and dinner. Plan this schedule including groceries. This way, you can prepare the recipes ahead of time; this will erase any meal-related disputes with the rest of the family and will not defeat the purpose of going vegan.

4. **Do Not Think Too Much About It**

Some people think this is more of something that society pushed you to do; hence, you start to think that this is a sacrifice, suffering, or something difficult. Remember that you are doing this because of personal conviction; more importantly, you are not doing this for someone else. You are doing this for yourself. Just enjoy it!

5. **Read More About Being a Vegan**

Knowledge is power. Knowing why being a vegan is beneficial, the more you will be motivated and dedicated and will increase your likelihood to stick to your new lifestyle. This will also result to better understanding of the lifestyle, will help you prepare even more and for you to know how to tweak the outlined details your read in books and internet about vegan, which can improve your learning curve.

6. **You Are Doing Something Mutually Beneficial**

   Remember, being a vegan means you are not just being good to yourself but to other stewards of this planet—the animals. So go ahead and reward yourself with a vegan treat occasionally.

7. **Never Think of Depriving Yourself**

   Do not focus on the food that you can't eat right away—eggs, milks, chicken, fish, etc.—because this will make things extra difficult to you. Instead, think of this as an opportunity to include new variations to your palate. The more options you have the easier it will be to remove those animal-based products from your menu. Depriving yourself at the early stages of the transition is the cause of the negative notions about vegan diet.

8. **Ask For Help**

While there is plethora of resources on the internet that can be helpful—from meal plans to tips—it is still best to consult a dietitian or nutritionist for expert advice. Remember, this diet is supposed to be beneficial and not detrimental. It is also best to do these consultations before you start the transition so you will be guided properly.

2d. Major Benefits of Going Vegan

One major question in going vegan is its health benefits. While it's true that a plant-based diet is beneficial in a lot of ways, the question is what are the major ones? In what way doing vegan diet can be considered as "the healthy way of living"?

One thing to bear in mind that, unlike meat eaters, vegetarians tend to eat less fatty food and in turn they take in more vitamins. As a result, they have lower intake of bad cholesterol in their bodies and would most likely have lower tendencies of developing chronic heart diseases.

However, scientific data are not adequate to support claims that vegan diet can be the key to a holistic healthy living because there are still other patterns and practices that each vegetarian would most likely follow, such as smoking, drinking, and lack of exercise. But here's what we know so far:

a. *Heart disease.* There are stunning evidences that suggest that vegetarians have lower risks of developing heart diseases by a large margin as compared to those who have meat-full diet. According to the Harvard Health Publication, "… a combined analysis of data from five prospective studies involving more than 76,000 participants published several years ago — vegetarians were, on average, 25% less likely to die of heart disease."

b. *Cancer.* While we can't really be sure for the rest of the degenerative diseases, one thing is for sure: eating lots of fruits and vegetables can reduce the risk of acquiring certain types of cancers. However, this does not mean that not having a plant-based diet can't decrease your likelihood of developing cancers. In an article published by Harvard Health Publication, they noted that a fish eater had a lower risk of certain cancer than a vegetarian does.

c. *Type 2 diabetes.* Plant-based diet have lesser starch content and by extension, can help the body in the production of insulin, which is very important in battling the risk of developing diabetes.

d. ***Bone health.*** Calcium is very important in bone development. The fear in going vegan is calcium deficiency because vegans would cut down the intake of milk and dairy products. However, certain vegetables can supply calcium including bok choy, broccoli, Chinese cabbage, collards, and kale.

Chapter Three: Vegan Recipes

Now that you are all set and ready to jump-start your vegan lifestyle, it is important to understand that your meal is the hero of this transition. Meals are very important to us human beings and there's no explaining why that is the case, it's quite obvious.

A plant-based diet is not big of a problem as these products are available all year long. You can even plant some on your garden or backyard for fresh harvest ingredients. Having a plant-based diet has many advantages as well, one of which is it is cost efficient. Vegetables are cheap and affordable as compared to meat and other animal-based products. In addition, that can be one motivation for you to become a vegan.

Crafted by some of known food bloggers — Erwan Heussaff, Stef Sanciano, Carmela Villegas-Agosta and Diane Nicole Go — below are recipes that you can prepare and can be included in your weekly meal schedule.

Erwan is a chef and entrepreneur who believes that food is an essential part in a healthy life. All his contents are available online at thefatkidinside.com.

Stef is a culinary arts graduate from Manila. She gained experience in the kitchens and restaurants of Singapore and is currently cooking up a storm in Jakarta.

Carmela's love for food started at a young age, fueled by her grandmother's cooking and food trip around the world. Eventually, she turned this passion and love into a business since 2011.

Diane is a graduate of the Ateneo de Manila University with a course in Legal Management and a minor in Creative Writing, she evaded the path of law to chase after food.

Richgail Enriquez also known as "RG", is a cook and a purveyor of recipes of both traditionally vegan and veganized Filipino dishes

Enjoy planning your vegan meals!

Green Soba Noodle Soup

Sometimes, we focus so much in food that are full in protein that we end up eating heavy. Hence, often times we just want to enjoy a bowl of hot soup that is oozing with flavor.

Ingredients:

1 portion of cha soba noodles

1 1/2 cup of boiling water

1/3 cup sliced scallions

1 green chili thinly sliced

3 tbsp soy sauce

1 tbsp miso paste

5 pieces of crunched up seaweed

1 tsp tahini or sesame paste

thai basil leaves

Instructions:

1. boil the soba noddles in the water for 3 mins.

2. Place in a bowl.

3. In the water, add the miso paste, soy sauce and tahini. Stir in until dissolve. Bring to a boil.

4. Place the soup on top of the noddles, ganish with the chili, thai basil and scallions.

Kimchi Brioche Pizza

Korean fusion dishes are pretty common these days. Kimchi, a popular Korean side dish, is in fact proving to be versatile and is slowly easing its way to Western palates. – Stef Sancianco

Ingredients:

2 slices of brioche loaf bread

6 strips bacon, sliced into small pieces

1/2 cup kimchi, chopped

2 tablespoons tomato sauce

1/2 cup grated mozzarella cheese

Optional toppings:

baby spinach

chopped Kale

spring onions

cilantro

Instructions:

Preheat oven to 350 deg F or 180 deg C. Once oven is hot, pre-bake the brioche slices for 3-5 minutes. Set aside.

In a pot, place the chopped bacon and slowly render the fat. Add in the chopped kimchi and continue to saute until the kimchi is slightly translucent. Optional ingredients to saute in are baby spinach or kale. Set aside once cooked.

28

To assemble, place the pre-baked slices of bread on a baking tray and spread 1 tablespoon tomato sauce on each. Sprinkle mozzarella cheese and then the kimchi and bacon mixture on top. Optional toppings to put are chopped herbs like fresh spring onions and/or cilantro to brighten up the dish.

Place in the oven and bake for 12-15 minutes or until melting and golden. For those who can take heat, serve with a drizzle of Sriracha sauce. Wait for a few minutes to cool down and enjoy!

Nutella-Raisin Bread Pudding

"Bread Pudding is a classic recipe that brings new life to your old bread. It is also very versatile from the bread choice to the toppings and to the custard filling." Says Carmela Villegas-Agosta

Ingredients:

Pudding

4 C Raisin Bread, sliced into cubes

2 ½ C Milk

¾ C Butter

2 eggs

½ C Brown Sugar

1 tsp Vanilla

½ C Peanut Butter or Nutella

Directions:

Grease your baking pan. Choose a baking pan that's at least 2 inches in height.

In a bowl, mix your milk, eggs, vanilla, ½ C melted butter and ¼ cup of sugar all together until well combined.

Place your raisin bread in your baking pan. Pour the milk-egg mixture onto the bread and let soak in the batter for about 15 minutes. Cut the remaining ¼ C butter into cubes and place around the bread. Spread peanut butter or hazelnut spread on top of the bread and sprinkle with the remaining sugar.

Place the pan in the oven at 180 C degrees for 30 minutes or until the custard cooks and the pudding becomes a nice golden color. Serve warm.

Before serving sprinkle some powdered sugar or serve with ice cream.

Vegan Filipino Peanut Stew, Kare-Kare

This dish, crafted by a Filipino cook, Richgail Enriquez, highlights a classic Filipino stew: the Kare-Kare. According to Richgail, "Filipinos often reserve this dish for big parties like town fiestas, christenings, even weddings. It's a dish that's both celebratory and celebrated."

This is the vegan version of this beloved Filipino dish.

Ingredients:

1 banana blossom bud, fresh (canned, which is ready to use, is an ok alternative)

3 tablespoons canola oil

4 garlic cloves, peeled, crushed, and minced

1 yellow onion, peeled and chopped

few pinches sea salt

6 cups water

2 eggplants, sliced

1 cup vegetable broth or more to taste

2-3 tablespoons achuete or annatto powder, fully dissolved in 2 cups water

1 cup peanuts, toasted and ground to a powder. (Peanut butter is an okay alternative).

½ cup white rice, toasted and ground to a powder, mixed in 1 cup water (make sure there are no lumps in the mixture)

1 small bunch long beans, cut to 2-inch slices, ends removed

2 pieces dried snow fungus, soaked in water for 1-3 minutes, cut into big chunks (textured soy protein is an ok alternative)

1 bundle bokchoy, washed, bottom stalk cut off (long bok choy is traditional but you may cut to chunks if preferred).

2 tablespoons black bean sauce mixed in 2 tablespoons seaweed flakes (as condiment)

Instructions:

Peel outer layers of banana blossom until you reach the pale pink, tender bud. Discard outer layers and yellow pistils or use as decor for plating. Have a large bowl of salt water nearby. Oil your knife and cutting board to prevent sap from sticking. Cut off stem and slice bud in half lengthwise. Cut in chunks and immediately submerge the banana blossom in salt water. Soak for at least 10 minutes. Discard soaking water and rinse thoroughly.

In a large pot, saute garlic with oil until fragrant. Follow with onions. Add few pinches of sea salt and saute until onions have turned soft and translucent.

Add banana blossom, eggplant, water, vegetable broth, and achuete mixture. Mix and cover pot. Simmer until eggplant and banana blossom are tender.

Mix in ground peanuts and rice mixture. Simmer for 10 minutes. If sauce gets too thick, add more water one cup at a time until consistency is creamy.

Adjust seasoning by adding more vegetable broth or ground peanuts to taste.

Add long beans, snow fungus, and bok choy. Put to a boil and turn off heat.

Serve hot preferably with rice and black bean condiment on the side.

Vegan Paella

Paella is a Valencian rice dish. Paella has ancient roots, but its modern form originated in the mid-19th century near Albufera lagoon on the east coast of Spain adjacent to the city of Valencia.

There are many versions of the Paella, and we are giving you Richgail's version of this dish. According to her, "Filipino style *Paella* is almost the same as the Spanish original except for some of the spices used. The Filipino version uses achuete or anatto powder as the food coloring instead of saffron threads...Some Filipino versions also use tomato sauce."

Ingredients:

3 tablespoons extra virgin olive oil

4 cloves of garlic, crushed

1 medium onion, chopped

2 roma tomatoes, chopped (preferably very ripe red)

1 small red bell pepper, sliced

1 teaspoon achuete or annatto powder (mixed in 3 tbsp water)

1 1/2 cup of rice (I used Eighth Wonder Kalinga Unoy)

2 cups warm water

1 cup of vegetable broth (I used the bouillon kind so I added more water)

1 can of straw mushrooms

1/2 cup of green peas, frozen and thawed

3 pcs bay leaves

a pinch of saffron threads

salt and pepper to taste (preferably sea salt and freshly ground pepper)

lemon wedges, for garnish

olives, for garnish (I used kalamata olives)

artichokes, for garnish (I used marinated artichoke hearts)

Directions:

1. In a skillet or shallow pan, saute the garlic with oil over medium heat.
2. Add the onions and tomatoes until fragrant and tender.
3. Add the red bell pepper and saute for another 5 minutes.
4. Pour in the rice grains, mix well making sure the grains are coated.
5. Add the water and vegetable broth, mixing well so the rice will have equal amounts of flavor. Simmer and occasionally mix for 5 minutes.

6. Top the rice with bay leaves and cover the pan. Let the rice cook for 15 minutes (no stirring).

7. Check the rice, if the top portion is still raw, add a little bit of water. Do this bit by bit and *gradually* until all liquid is absorbed and the rice is fully cooked.

8. Once the rice is cooked, mix in the peas, saffron threads, and achioete/annatto mixture.

9. Add salt and pepper to taste. Simmer for about 5 minutes. Turn off the heat.

10. Add the artichokes, olives, and lemons on top as garnish.

11. Serve hot.

Tart Gaspacho with Herb Parmesan Salad

Ingredients:

For the Gazpacho

5 big tomatoes

1 large cucumber

1 red pepper

1 green pepper

1/2 cup of day old bread chopped

5 tablespoons of red wine vingear

3 garlic cloves chopped

3/4 cup Extra Virgin Olive Oil

Salt and Pepper To taste

For the Garnish

per dish

a pinch of flat leaf parsley

1 tsp of lemon rind

1 tbsp of parmesan cheese

1 tbsp of sour cream

a pinch of salt

(optional) yellow baby tomatoes sliced, red onion and cucumber shavings

Instructions:

Blend all the chopped and cleaned vegetables together. Once soup like add the bread, the vinegar and slowly trickle in the olive oil while blending. Salt and pepper to taste. For the toppings, leave the parsley whole, mix with the other ingredients. Place on the soup with a dollop of sour cream and salt. Use optional garnish to make it look more intricate.

Fresh Lumpia

Lumpia is a fried spring roll and is very common in Indonesia and the Philippines. It is a snack made of thin dough wrapping called "lumpia wrapper" and is filled with chopped vegetables like carrots, cabbages, green beans, and either ground chicken and pork. The vegan version goes perfectly well with a tofu.

In the Philippines, however, there is a different version of this savoury snack and it's called "fresh lumpia".

Ingredients:

For the Filling:

3 tablespoons canola oil

3 garlic cloves, peeled, crushed, and minced

1 yellow onion, peeled and chopped

1 cup thinly sliced green beans, ends discarded

1 cup shredded cabbage

1 cup bean sprouts

1 cup chickpeas from can (save the brine)

1 cup diced jicama

1 cup diced carrots

1 cup diced potatoes

1 cup diced sweet potatoes

1 cup diced extra firm tofu

15-20 pieces lettuce leaves, washed and thoroughly dried

few pinches sea salt

2-3 tablespoons organic brown sugar

2-3 tablespoons crushed peanuts for garnish (optional)

For the Sauce:

2 cups water

3-4 tablespoons soy sauce

¼ cup organic brown sugar

4 tablespoons potato starch, dissolved and mixed in ¼ cup of water

3 garlic cloves,peeled, crushed, and minced (optional)

For the Wrapper/Crepe:

½ cup unbleached flour

1 cup non-dairy milk

½ cup chickpea brine

1 teaspoon canola oil

Instructions:

For the Filling:

1. Heat a medium pan over medium heat and saute onions and garlic with oil until onions have turned translucent.

2. Add potatoes and sweet potatoes and cook until they have softened. Add a little bit of water if needed to deglaze the pan.

3. Meanwhile, fry tofu on a separate pan over high heat until golden brown.

4. Once potatoes are tender, add carrots and jicama and cook until they have softened.

5. Add green beans, chickpeas, and bean sprouts.

6. Place fried tofu to the filling. Thoroughly mix and cook for another 5 minutes.

7. Season with salt and brown sugar.

8. Turn off heat and set aside.

For the Sauce:

1. Pour water to a small sauce pan or pot and heat over low to medium heat.

2. Pour soy sauce and brown sugar.

3. Mix potato starch mixture/slurry and keep mixing until creamy.

4. Add garlic and cook for another 2-3 minutes. (optional)

5. Turn off heat and set aside.

For the Wrapper:

1. Using a bowl, whisk together flour, milk, and chickpea brine.

2. Heat a nonstick pan over low heat. Once hot enough, pour a little bit of oil.

3. Turn down heat to low heat and lift up pan away from the heat. Pour a thin layer of batter and immediately swirl pan around to create a thin crepe.

4. Put down pan and cook for 3-5 minutes or until crepe is no longer sticking to the pan.

5. Using a thin metal spatula or ladle, flip crepe to cook the other side.

6. Repeat steps to make multiple crepes.

7. Alternatively, you could go with ready-to-use Vietnamese rice paper for a gluten-free option.

To Assemble:

1. Place lettuce on the middle of the wrapper and place a spoonful of filling on top of the lettuce.

2. Roll wrapper from one side to the other. Halfway into it, fold the lower part then continue rolling. The top part should be where the lettuce leaves are sticking out.

3. Repeat steps until everything is rolled.

4. Top rolls with sauce and crushed peanuts.

5. Serve immediately.

Vegan Filipino Spaghetti

One of the beloved dishes in the world is spaghetti, and this dish could be one of those you can kiss goodbye once you decide to go vegan. But no worries, with this vegan version you can kiss those fingers again and say *delicioso!*

INGREDIENTS

For the "meat" of the sauce:

- 12 ounces extra-firm tofu, frozen overnight or for at least 4 hours, then thawed, then crumbled (using your hands or food processor)
- vegan hotdogs, thinly sliced
- 4-5 tablespoons canola oil
- 3-5 tablespoons refined coconut oil

For the sauce:

- 5 cloves garlic, peeled, crushed, and minced
- 1 cup roughly chopped yellow onion
- 1 cup roughly chopped celery sticks
- 1 cup roughly chopped carrots

- ½ cup roughly chopped, red bell pepper, seeds removed
- pinch of salt
- pinch of pepper
- 1 tablespoon tomato paste
- 1 tablespoon sweet pickle relish
- ¼ cup maple syrup (agave or regular natural sugar works too)
- 3-4 tablespoons soy sauce
- ¼ cup non-dairy milk
- cups tomato sauce

For the noodles:

- 1 pound Spaghetti pasta
- medium size pot of hot water

For garnish: (optional)

- ¼ cup grated vegan cheddar cheese as topping (optional)

Instructions:

1 Heat medium size pan over high heat. Once hot, pour oil until it covers the base of the pan. Wait until oil is very hot. Carefully add crumbled tofu (do not overcrowd the pan)

and fry until tofu is golden brown on all sides. Transfer to a plate.

2   Using the same pan, fry hotdog slices and sprinkle sugar and salt. Fry both sides and turn off heat. Transfer alongside fried tofu.

3   Place onions, celery, bell pepper, and carrots in a food processor and pulse for one minute or until finely minced. Transfer to a bowl.

4   Using the same pan you fried the tofu and hotdogs on, saute garlic until light golden. Follow with finely minced vegetables, salt, and pepper. Stir and cook for 3-5 minutes.

5   Add tomato sauce, tomato paste, sweet relish, soy sauce, maple syrup, and non-dairy milk. Mix well, cover, and simmer for 5 minutes, stirring every minute so sauce won't stick on the bottom of the pan.

6   Add fried tofu and hotdogs. Mix well and if desired, add more salt and pepper to taste. Simmer for another 5 minutes, stirring occasionally. Turn off heat.

7   Cook spaghetti per package's direction (usually 1 lb of spaghetti in 4 quarts of boiling pot of water) until pasta is tender. Drain well using a colander.

8   To serve, place sauce over noodles and top with grated vegan cheese. Serve warm.

Chapter Four: Keeping It Real

Obesity, heart diseases, diabetes and cancers—the facts are speaking for themselves, these are still the number one killers of men and women across the board. However, we all can deviate from these; prevent them at the least by doing something good for ourselves and our fellow tenants in this planet.

If you ate still unsure if you want to follow this diet, below are some fact-rich talking points to consider.

1. Just like starting on a new hobby, this change in your lifestyle will require you forming a community with people of the same interest. This is because support is essential in making it through this change.

2. Being a vegan does not stop once you start doing it. You have to understand that, aside from your personal reasons, health reasons and perhaps religious reasons, becoming vegan constitute a binding to protect animal welfare. It would be best to write something about your experiences in becoming a vegan, how it affected your health and your body holistically. This will not only serve as a testimonial for others to understand plant-based diet, but this will also raise awareness.

3. You are also doing something for the next generation. Raising animals for meat is a leading factor to global warming. Producing those juicy meats require a large volume of clean water, and often than not, factories abuse the environment by throwing its waste products back to where they got their materials: environment. Having a plant-based diet can reduce these detrimental factors by large, and by extension, saving our planet for the next generation.

4. Remember that most vegan food are cheap. Eating an inexpensive meal means more savings in the bank, which at the end of the day, means a lot to anyone.

5. You will be at par with notable individuals like Chris Campbell, Ken Bradshaw, Ellen Degeneres, Tobey Maguire, Alanis Morissette, and Ginnifer Goodwin.

6. Vegan diet possess indicative health benefits with the fact that your meal contains less toxins and drugs. R raised in densely compressed areas, animals are sprayed with pesticides and other animal maintenance, which is important for their survival. These chemicals are then carried over to the meat we eat once these animals are slaughtered and turned to meat products.

7. In relation to point 6, fresh fruits and vegetables contain phytochemicals, minerals, vitamins, enzymes and fiber, which are essential to bodily development.

8. Of course, let us be real that having little intake of fats means slender and sexier body. In addition, it is true that maintaining a healthy weight is lot easier done with a vegan diet.

9. For age conscious individuals, while this is considered a myth, but keeping a plant-based diet is believed to slow aging.

10. For adults who are prone to chronic constipation, having a plant-based diet can ease out bowel movement due to the considerable number of fiber present in fresh fruits and vegetables.

Conclusion

It is imperative to understand that vegan diet might or might not work out for some of us. We adapt to a certain lifestyle pattern due to various reasons — health, political views, personal conviction — and we follow them in such a way that is easy and practical. Nevertheless, it is also important to understand that regardless of the benefits highlighted in this reading materials that are associated with vegan-based diet, having a healthy body is not entirely linked with having a plant-based diet.

Diet is just one factor to consider in evaluating one's health, as this is a factor for experts to understand how we treat our body. Experts would highly suggest that when there's a change of lifestyle, there should also be adjustments to one's routines.

While majority of the vegetarians are proving to be healthy due to the correct practices in their chosen lifestyle, some are not. This is because other practices are still present regardless of this chosen one like smoking, excessive drinking, and more specifically, lack of proper exercises.

Moreover, some people decide to agree that vegan diet is the easiest way to lose the belly fats, achieve that model-like body, and this is fairly true. There are many testimonials on the internet that will show you their transformation after following a rigorous set of workouts and a strict diet. Beyoncé followed a 22 day meal plan to get back on shape, as previously reported. You can also check Erwan Heussaf's website, thefatkidinside.com, for other related testimonials.

Finally, any change in lifestyle is, usually, not good when it is done overnight. This change, much like going in a battle, should be carefully planned, must be studied, and be done with an open mind. Most people who tried doing this change in lifestyle did not see it through because of lack of education and setting of false expectations. Experts say to take this change easy, never be restrictive on the early stages of the transition, and have a total dedication. It is also highly advised to seek for experts' advice.

Becoming a vegan can be dangerous if done incorrectly, but if done otherwise, can be a source of mutual support and mutually exclusive benefits.

Bibliography

Babauta, L. (n.d.). *HOW TO DO THE CHALLENGE THE EASY WAY*. Retrieved from 7DAY VEGAN: http://7dayvegan.com/easy/

Becoming a vegetarian. (2009, 2016, October, March). Retrieved from Harvard Health Publication: http://www.health.harvard.edu/staying-healthy/becoming-a-vegetarian

Development, T. O.-o. (2017). *Obesity Update 2017.*

Enriquez, R. (2012, May 18). *VEGAN PAELLA, FILIPINO STYLE*. Retrieved from Astig Vegan: http://www.astigvegan.com/vegan-paella-filipino-style/

Enriquez, R. (2015, June). *LUMPIANG SARIWA RECIPE*. Retrieved from Astig Vegan: http://www.astigvegan.com/lumpiang-sariwa-recipe/

Enriquez, R. (2015, December). *VEGAN FILIPINO SPAGHETTI*. Retrieved from Astig Vegan: http://www.astigvegan.com/vegan-filipino-spaghetti/

Enriquez, R. (2017, May 13). *VEGAN FILIPINO PEANUT STEW, KARE-KARE, WITH VIDEO*. Retrieved from Astig Vegan: http://www.astigvegan.com/vegan-kare-kare-recipe-with-video/

Heussaff, E. (2012, November 13). *TART GASPACHO WITH HERB PARMESAN SALAD*. Retrieved from The Fat Kid Inside: http://www.thefatkidinside.com/healthy-lifestyles/tart-gaspacho-with-herb-parmesan-salad

Heussaff, E. (2016, November 18). *GREEN SOBA NOODLE SOUP*. Retrieved from The Fat Kid Inside: http://www.thefatkidinside.com/recipe/green-soba-noodle-soup

Sancianco, S. (2016, July 28). *5-INGREDIENT RECIPE: KIMCHI BRIOCHE PIZZA*. Retrieved from The Fat Kid Inside:

http://www.thefatkidinside.com/recipe/5-ingredient-recipe-kimchi-brioche-pizza

Stevens, K. (2014, May 10). *No Lie Can Live Forever: Predicting a Vegan America by 2050*. Retrieved from Huffington Post: http://www.huffingtonpost.com/kathy-stevens/predicting-a-vegan-america_b_4905691.html

Two-Week Vegan Meal Plan. (n.d.). Retrieved from PETA: https://www.peta.org/living/food/two-week-vegan-meal-plan/

Villegas-Agosta, C. (2016, October 24). *NUTELLA-RAISIN BREAD PUDDING*. Retrieved from The Fat Kid Inside: http://www.thefatkidinside.com/recipe/nutella-raisin-bread-pudding